BARRETTE ESOPHAGUS
CAUSES
Including (GERD)

*In-Depth Resource for Managing Barrette
Esophagus with Early Intervention, Dietary
Changes, and Support Strategies*

Cormac Cristiano

Disclaimer

This book, *Barrette Esophagus Causes - Including (GERD): In-Depth Resource For Managing Barrette Esophagus With Early Intervention, Dietary Changes, And Support Strategies*, is intended for informational and educational purposes only. It is not a substitute for professional medical advice, diagnosis, or treatment. Always consult a qualified healthcare provider with any questions or concerns you may have regarding your health or a medical condition.

The information presented in this book is based on research, available resources, and the author understands at the time of writing. However, medical knowledge and recommendations evolve over time, and the author does not guarantee the accuracy, completeness, or timeliness of the information contained within. Readers are encouraged to use this book as a general guide and to seek updated advice from healthcare professionals before making any decisions related to their health.

The author does not endorse any specific individuals, products, websites, organizations, or other entities mentioned in this book. Any references to external names, entities, or products are for informational purposes only and do not constitute an endorsement or recommendation. The author assumes no liability for any outcomes, decisions, or actions taken based on the information in this book.

By reading this book, you agree to assume full responsibility for any use of the information provided and to release the author from any liability related to personal health decisions or outcomes.

About This Book

The book titled *Barrett's Esophagus Causes: An In-Depth Resource for Managing Barrett's Esophagus with Early Intervention, Dietary Changes, and Support Strategies* serves as a vital guide for individuals navigating the complexities of Barrett's Esophagus and its association with gastroesophageal reflux disease (GERD). This comprehensive resource not only elucidates the condition itself, but also underscores the critical link between GERD and Barrett's Esophagus, highlighting the importance of early intervention and proactive lifestyle modifications. Readers will gain insights into how this guide aims to empower them to manage their condition effectively, fostering a sense of agency and encouraging them to take charge of their health.

A key focus of this resource is the pivotal role that diet and lifestyle play in the management of Barrett's Esophagus. The text elaborates on how dietary choices can significantly impact esophageal health, guiding readers toward making informed decisions about their nutrition. With a commitment to enhancing readers' understanding of their condition, the guide provides a structured overview of essential content, ensuring easy navigation through complex topics. Furthermore, it emphasizes the necessity of support strategies and medical guidance, reassuring readers that they are not alone on this journey and that resources are available for ongoing education and support.

Understanding Barrett's Esophagus requires familiarity with its definition, symptoms, and the diagnostic processes involved. The book outlines the symptoms associated with Barrett's Esophagus, emphasizing the critical need for early detection and regular monitoring. It dispels common misconceptions surrounding the condition while also discussing risk factors and potential complications that can arise if left untreated. By presenting current research and findings, the book equips readers with a robust foundation for understanding their health.

Exploring the causes and risk factors associated with Barrett's Esophagus, the text delves into the multifaceted nature of the condition. It examines the relationship between GERD and Barrett's Esophagus while considering other contributors, such as obesity, smoking, and genetic predispositions. The book further emphasizes the importance of recognizing individual risk factors and lifestyle influences on esophageal health, enabling readers to adopt preventive strategies tailored to their unique circumstances.

Dietary changes play a central role in the management of Barrett's Esophagus, and the book provides detailed guidance on nutritional choices. By outlining beneficial foods, those to avoid, and meal planning strategies, the text serves as a practical tool for individuals seeking to enhance their dietary habits. It highlights the significance of hydration and offers tips for adapting recipes and dining out safely, ultimately aiming to foster a positive relationship with food and nutrition.

In addition to dietary considerations, the book emphasizes the necessity of a support network, encompassing family, friends, and support groups. It underscores the value of psychological support and effective communication with healthcare providers, guiding readers in setting realistic health goals and managing anxiety. Through resources for ongoing support and education, the book nurtures a sense of community and shared experiences, promoting resilience in the face of health challenges.

Recognizing the importance of early intervention and regular monitoring, the book elaborates on the frequency of check-ups and the role of diagnostic procedures such as biopsies. It emphasizes esophageal cancer awareness and the benefits of proactive treatment interventions, ensuring that readers are informed about their options. By fostering a clear understanding of treatment plans and the significance of adhering to medical advice, the guide empowers readers to advocate for their health.

Lifestyle modifications are also explored, with an emphasis on weight management, smoking cessation, and stress reduction techniques. The book discusses the impact of alcohol consumption and the importance of sleep quality, encouraging readers to adopt sustainable lifestyle changes that support their overall well-being. By incorporating physical activities and hobbies that promote health, readers are inspired to create a healthier living environment.

The resource also addresses potential complications associated with Barrett's Esophagus, underscoring the importance of recognizing warning signs that necessitate immediate medical attention. It provides strategies for managing acute symptoms and emphasizes the role of nutrition in recovery from complications, ensuring that readers are well-prepared for any challenges they may face.

In summary, *Barrett's Esophagus Causes* is an essential resource that not only enhances understanding of Barrett's Esophagus and its connection to GERD but also equips readers with practical strategies for managing their condition. With a focus on dietary changes, lifestyle modifications, and the significance of support networks, this guide is an invaluable tool for anyone seeking to navigate the complexities of Barrett's Esophagus with confidence and knowledge.

Table of Contents

Introduction Headings

Overview of Barrett's Esophagus and Its Significance

Barrett's Esophagus is a condition where the tissue lining the esophagus changes, often due to prolonged exposure to stomach acid. This alteration can increase the risk of esophageal cancer, making it crucial to monitor and manage. Understanding this condition is the first step toward effective management and prevention of more severe complications.

Recognizing Barrett's Esophagus early allows for timely intervention and better outcomes. Patients should be aware of symptoms such as difficulty swallowing, heartburn, and regurgitation, as these may indicate an underlying issue that requires further evaluation by a healthcare professional.

The Connection Between GERD and Barrett's Esophagus

Gastroesophageal reflux disease (GERD) is a chronic condition where stomach acid frequently flows back into the esophagus, causing irritation and inflammation. Over time, this chronic irritation can lead to Barrett's Esophagus. Therefore, individuals with persistent GERD symptoms are at a higher risk for developing this condition, emphasizing the need for effective management of acid reflux.

To prevent Barrett's Esophagus, it is essential to address GERD symptoms proactively. This can involve lifestyle changes such as avoiding trigger foods, maintaining a healthy weight, and possibly using medications prescribed by a healthcare provider to manage acid reflux.

Importance of Early Intervention and Lifestyle Changes

Early intervention is critical in managing Barrett's Esophagus and preventing complications. Regular monitoring through endoscopy allows healthcare providers to assess the condition of the esophagus and detect any changes early. If Barrett's is diagnosed, treatment plans may include medication, lifestyle modifications, or more invasive procedures if necessary.

Implementing lifestyle changes can significantly improve symptoms and quality of life. This includes maintaining a balanced diet, avoiding foods that trigger reflux, elevating the head during sleep, and quitting smoking, all of which can help reduce acid exposure and lower the risk of progression.

How This Guide Will Help You Manage Your Condition

This guide provides practical strategies for managing Barrett's Esophagus effectively. It outlines key dietary modifications, such as incorporating alkaline foods, reducing spicy and acidic items, and focusing on whole grains, fruits, and vegetables. These dietary changes can help soothe the esophagus and minimize reflux episodes.

Additionally, the guide emphasizes the importance of regular follow-ups with healthcare professionals to monitor the condition. It also includes tips on how to communicate effectively with your healthcare team, ensuring that you receive personalized care and support throughout your management journey.

Encouragement for Proactive Health Management

Proactive health management is vital for individuals with Barrett's Esophagus. By staying informed and engaged in their care, patients can take charge of their health and make decisions that positively impact their condition. This includes understanding the importance of medication adherence and recognizing when to seek further evaluation.

Encouragement to adopt a supportive community can also enhance management efforts. Joining support groups or seeking out resources can provide valuable insights and motivation, helping individuals stay committed to their health journey and improve their overall well-being.

The Role of Diet and Lifestyle in Barrett's Esophagus Management

Understanding the Impact of Diet on Esophageal Health

Diet plays a crucial role in maintaining esophageal health, particularly for individuals with Barrett's Esophagus. Foods that are high in acid, spicy, or fatty can trigger gastroesophageal reflux disease (GERD) symptoms, leading to increased irritation of the esophagus lining. It's essential to identify these trigger foods through a food diary, allowing individuals to understand how their diet affects their symptoms.

To promote healing and reduce symptoms, focus on a diet rich in whole foods, including fruits, vegetables, whole grains, and lean proteins. Incorporating alkaline foods, such as bananas and melons, can help neutralize stomach acid. It's also beneficial to eat smaller, more frequent meals and avoid lying down immediately after eating to minimize reflux.

Importance of Support Strategies and Medical Guidance

Navigating Barrett's Esophagus requires a comprehensive approach that includes both medical guidance and supportive strategies. Regular check-ups with a healthcare provider are essential for monitoring the condition and discussing any new symptoms or dietary challenges. This proactive communication helps tailor treatment plans and ensures early intervention when necessary.

Support strategies can include joining support groups or engaging in community resources where individuals can share experiences and coping strategies. It's helpful to discuss lifestyle changes, such as weight management or quitting smoking, with healthcare professionals who can provide tailored advice and encouragement for lasting change.

Overview of the Content Structure for Easy Navigation

To effectively manage Barrett's Esophagus, having a structured approach to the information is vital. This guide is divided into clear sections that address dietary modifications, lifestyle changes, and medical management strategies. Each section builds on the previous one, providing a logical flow of information that makes it easier for readers to follow.

Navigating through the content should be intuitive. Headings and subheadings are used consistently to highlight key points, and bullet points or lists are incorporated for quick reference. This structured layout helps readers quickly find the information they need without feeling overwhelmed.

Commitment to Making Informed Dietary Choices

Making informed dietary choices is crucial for managing Barrett's Esophagus effectively. This involves learning to read food labels carefully and understanding how ingredients can affect esophageal health. Begin by eliminating processed foods that contain additives and preservatives, which can exacerbate symptoms.

To ensure dietary choices are beneficial, consider meal prepping to control ingredients and portion sizes. Planning meals around low-acid and anti-inflammatory foods can enhance compliance and make healthier eating more manageable. Keeping a list of safe and unsafe foods can further aid decision-making, simplifying the process of meal selection.

Resources for Ongoing Support and Education

Accessing reliable resources for ongoing support and education is vital for individuals managing Barrett's Esophagus. Numerous organizations provide information on the latest research, dietary guidelines, and coping strategies. Online platforms, such as forums and webinars, can connect individuals with experts and peers who understand the challenges of living with this condition.

Local support groups or community health organizations often host educational events, providing opportunities to learn and share experiences. Staying engaged with these resources fosters a sense of community and empowers individuals to make informed decisions about their health and dietary choices.

CHAPTER 1:

What is Barrett's Esophagus?

Definition and Explanation of Barrett's Esophagus

Barrett's Esophagus is a condition where the tissue lining the esophagus changes, often due to long-term exposure to stomach acid. This condition involves the replacement of normal squamous cells with columnar cells, a process called intestinal metaplasia. This transformation is significant because it can increase the risk of developing esophageal cancer. Understanding this condition is essential for effective management and treatment.

Management of Barrett's Esophagus typically involves monitoring the condition and making lifestyle changes to reduce symptoms. Patients may need to undergo regular endoscopic examinations to check for precancerous changes. Recognizing

Barrett's Esophagus early can help in implementing preventive measures and ensuring timely medical intervention.

Connection to Gastroesophageal Reflux Disease (GERD)

Gastroesophageal reflux disease (GERD) is a major risk factor for Barrett's Esophagus. GERD occurs when stomach acid frequently flows back into the esophagus, leading to inflammation and damage over time. Chronic acid exposure can trigger the cellular changes seen in Barrett's Esophagus. Understanding this connection is crucial for patients experiencing persistent heartburn or acid reflux symptoms.

To manage GERD effectively, individuals can make lifestyle changes such as avoiding trigger foods, eating smaller meals, and not lying down immediately after eating. Over-the-counter antacids or prescription medications may also be recommended to reduce stomach acid and alleviate symptoms. Addressing GERD early can help prevent the progression to Barrett's Esophagus.

Symptoms Associated with Barrett's Esophagus

The symptoms of Barrett's Esophagus often overlap with those of GERD, including heartburn, difficulty swallowing, and a sensation of food being stuck in the throat. However, some patients may experience atypical symptoms such as chest pain or cough. It is important to monitor these symptoms closely, especially if they worsen over time.

To manage symptoms effectively, patients should keep a journal of their food intake and symptom patterns. This record can help identify trigger foods and activities that worsen symptoms. Simple dietary adjustments, such as reducing spicy or acidic foods and increasing hydration, can also provide relief.

How Barrett's Esophagus is Diagnosed

Barrett's Esophagus is typically diagnosed through an upper endoscopy, where a thin, flexible tube with a camera is inserted into the esophagus to visualize and obtain tissue samples. During the procedure, the doctor may perform a biopsy to check for cellular changes indicative of Barrett's Esophagus. This process is essential for an accurate diagnosis.

Patients may need to prepare for the endoscopy by fasting for a specified period. After the procedure, it is common to experience some throat discomfort, but recovery is usually quick. Follow-up appointments are important to discuss biopsy results and any necessary treatment plans.

Importance of Early Detection

Early detection of Barrett's Esophagus is vital because it allows for timely intervention and management. Identifying the condition before it progresses to dysplasia or esophageal cancer can significantly improve outcomes. Regular monitoring and screenings for individuals with chronic GERD symptoms are recommended to catch any changes early.

To promote early detection, patients should discuss their GERD symptoms with their healthcare providers and consider regular endoscopies as advised. Being proactive about gastrointestinal health can lead to better management and prevention of serious complications.

Risk Factors for Developing Barrett's Esophagus

Several risk factors can increase the likelihood of developing Barrett's Esophagus, including chronic GERD, obesity, smoking, and age (typically over 50). Men are also more likely to develop this condition than women. Understanding these risk factors can help individuals take preventive measures.

Managing risk factors involves adopting a healthy lifestyle, such as maintaining a healthy weight, quitting smoking, and engaging in regular physical activity. Dietary changes, such as increasing fruits and vegetables while reducing processed foods, can also support esophageal health.

Potential Complications if Left Untreated

If Barrett's Esophagus is left untreated, it can lead to serious complications, including high-grade dysplasia and esophageal adenocarcinoma (a type of cancer). These complications can be life-threatening and require aggressive treatment. Early intervention is key to preventing progression.

Patients should be aware of the importance of routine monitoring and follow-ups with their healthcare providers. By addressing Barrett's Esophagus early, individuals can reduce the risk of complications and improve their overall quality of life.

Differences Between Barrett's Esophagus and GERD

While Barrett's Esophagus and GERD are connected, they are not the same condition. GERD is characterized by frequent acid reflux, leading to symptoms such as heartburn, while Barrett's Esophagus involves structural changes in the esophagus due to prolonged acid exposure. Understanding these differences is crucial for effective management.

Management strategies for GERD include dietary modifications, lifestyle changes, and medications. In contrast, Barrett's Esophagus may require additional monitoring and treatment options, including endoscopies and potential surgery if dysplasia is detected. Recognizing the distinction between these conditions aids in appropriate treatment.

Importance of Regular Monitoring

Regular monitoring of Barrett's Esophagus is essential to detect any changes in the cells lining the esophagus and to manage the risk of esophageal cancer. This often involves periodic endoscopies and biopsies as determined by a healthcare provider. Consistent monitoring can lead to early detection of any precancerous changes, allowing for timely intervention.

Patients should establish a schedule for follow-up appointments with their healthcare providers, who will determine the appropriate frequency of monitoring based on individual risk factors. Adhering to this schedule can help patients stay informed about their condition and take proactive steps toward management.

Common Misconceptions About Barrett's Esophagus

One common misconception about Barrett's Esophagus is that it only affects older adults or those with severe GERD symptoms. In reality, younger individuals can also be diagnosed with the condition, especially if they have chronic acid reflux. Educating oneself about Barrett's Esophagus is crucial for understanding its risks and symptoms.

Another misconception is that Barrett's Esophagus always leads to cancer. While it does increase the risk, not all patients with Barrett's Esophagus will develop esophageal cancer. Regular monitoring and lifestyle modifications can significantly reduce this risk. Educating oneself can empower patients to seek timely care and support.

Signs That Indicate a Need for Medical Evaluation

Certain signs should prompt individuals to seek medical evaluation, including persistent heartburn, difficulty swallowing, unexplained weight loss, or persistent cough. These symptoms may indicate a worsening condition that requires immediate attention. Early evaluation can lead to timely diagnosis and intervention.

Patients should not ignore these symptoms or assume they are just part of aging or dietary indiscretion. If symptoms persist or worsen, contacting a healthcare provider is essential to ensure appropriate evaluation and management of potential underlying conditions.

The Role of Endoscopy in Diagnosis

Endoscopy plays a crucial role in the diagnosis of Barrett's Esophagus. During the procedure, a flexible tube with a camera is used to visualize the esophagus and assess any changes in the lining. Biopsies may be taken to confirm the presence of Barrett's Esophagus and check for dysplasia.

Patients may be anxious about the procedure, but understanding the process can help alleviate concerns. The preparation typically involves fasting, and sedation is usually provided for comfort. Post-procedure, patients can expect guidance on follow-up care based on the findings.

Current Research and Findings Related to Barrett's Esophagus

Current research on Barrett's Esophagus focuses on understanding the disease's mechanisms, risk factors, and potential treatments. Studies are investigating the genetic and environmental influences on the development of Barrett's Esophagus and its progression to esophageal cancer.

This ongoing research aims to improve patient outcomes and inform better management strategies.

Staying informed about the latest research findings is essential for patients and healthcare providers alike. Engaging with support groups and educational resources can help individuals understand new developments in Barrett's Esophagus and its management.

CHAPTER 2:

Causes and Risk Factors

Detailed Look at GERD and Its Relation to Barrett's Esophagus

Gastroesophageal reflux disease (GERD) is a chronic condition characterized by the backflow of stomach acids into the esophagus. This acid exposure can damage the esophageal lining and lead to complications such as Barrett's Esophagus, a condition where the cells lining the esophagus undergo changes due to persistent irritation. Understanding GERD is crucial as it serves as the primary risk factor for developing Barrett's Esophagus; effectively managing GERD through lifestyle modifications and medications can significantly reduce the risk of progression.

To manage GERD, individuals can adopt several practical strategies, such as eating smaller meals and avoiding trigger foods like spicy or acidic items. Elevating the head during sleep and avoiding lying down immediately after meals can also help reduce acid reflux episodes. Regular consultations with healthcare providers to discuss symptoms and adjust treatment plans as necessary are vital in preventing Barrett's Esophagus.

Other Potential Causes (e.g., Obesity, Smoking)

Obesity and smoking are significant lifestyle factors that can exacerbate GERD symptoms and increase the risk of Barrett's Esophagus. Excess body weight can put pressure on the stomach, leading to more frequent acid reflux episodes. Smoking, on the other hand, can weaken the lower esophageal sphincter, allowing stomach acids to escape into the esophagus more easily. Both conditions are modifiable, making it essential to address them as part of a comprehensive health management plan.

To combat obesity, individuals can focus on maintaining a balanced diet rich in fruits, vegetables, and whole grains while incorporating regular physical activity into their routine. Smoking cessation is equally crucial; utilizing resources such as support groups or cessation programs can significantly enhance the likelihood of quitting, ultimately reducing the risk of Barrett's Esophagus.

Genetic Factors and Family History

Genetic predisposition and family history play a notable role in the development of Barrett's Esophagus. Individuals with a family history of the condition or related diseases, such as esophageal cancer, may have a higher likelihood of developing Barrett's Esophagus themselves. This genetic link underscores the importance of understanding personal health history and sharing it with healthcare providers for appropriate screening and preventive measures.

For individuals with a family history of Barrett's Esophagus, proactive monitoring and regular check-ups are essential. Discussing family health history during medical consultations can help healthcare professionals assess risk factors and recommend timely screenings, enabling early intervention if needed.

Role of Diet in Exacerbating Symptoms

Diet significantly influences GERD symptoms and, consequently, the risk of developing Barrett's Esophagus. Certain foods and beverages, such as caffeine, alcohol, chocolate, and fatty meals, can relax the lower esophageal sphincter, leading to increased acid reflux. Adopting a diet that minimizes these trigger foods can help manage GERD symptoms and reduce the risk of Barrett's Esophagus progression.

Individuals should consider keeping a food diary to identify personal triggers and adjust their diet accordingly. Incorporating a diet rich in anti-inflammatory foods like leafy greens, whole grains, and lean proteins while avoiding processed and fried foods can create a more favorable environment for esophageal health

The Importance of Understanding Individual Risk Factors

Recognizing individual risk factors for Barrett's Esophagus is essential for effective management and prevention. Each person may have different combinations of risk factors, including lifestyle choices, medical history, and genetic predisposition. Understanding these factors can empower individuals to take proactive steps to mitigate their risks.

Assessing personal risk factors involves reflecting on lifestyle habits, such as diet, exercise, and smoking status, as well as considering family medical history. Consulting with healthcare professionals can provide personalized insights and recommendations, enabling individuals to tailor their prevention strategies effectively.

Environmental Influences on Esophageal Health

Environmental factors, such as exposure to certain chemicals or pollutants, can impact esophageal health and contribute to the development of Barrett's Esophagus. Studies suggest that occupational hazards, such as exposure to harmful substances, may increase the risk of GERD and Barrett's Esophagus. Recognizing these influences is essential for adopting preventive measures.

Individuals can reduce environmental risks by being aware of their surroundings and minimizing exposure to known irritants. This might involve using protective equipment in occupational settings or choosing products that do not contain harmful chemicals at home. Promoting a healthy living environment can contribute to overall esophageal health.

The Impact of Age on Barrett's Esophagus Development

Age is a significant factor in the development of Barrett's Esophagus, with the risk increasing as individuals get older. This trend may be due to the cumulative effects of long-term GERD and other lifestyle factors over time. Understanding the connection between age and esophageal health is crucial for timely interventions and screenings.

To manage age-related risks, individuals should engage in regular health screenings and communicate any symptoms to their healthcare providers. Maintaining a healthy lifestyle through balanced nutrition, regular exercise, and avoiding smoking can also help mitigate the effects of aging on esophageal health.

Gender Differences in Barrett's Esophagus Prevalence

Research indicates that Barrett's Esophagus is more prevalent in men than in women. This disparity may be attributed to biological differences, hormonal influences, or variations in lifestyle factors. Understanding these differences is vital for tailoring prevention strategies and health interventions based on gender.

Men can focus on specific risk reduction strategies, such as maintaining a healthy weight, managing stress, and avoiding smoking. Women should also be mindful of their risk factors and engage in regular screenings, particularly if they have a history of GERD or other related conditions.

The Role of Medications in Managing GERD

Medications play a crucial role in managing GERD and preventing its progression to Barrett's Esophagus. Common treatments include proton pump inhibitors (PPIs) and H2 receptor antagonists, which reduce stomach acid production and alleviate symptoms. Understanding the appropriate use of these medications is essential for effective management.

Individuals should work closely with their healthcare providers to determine the best medication regimen for their specific needs. Regular follow-ups can help assess the effectiveness of treatment and make necessary adjustments, ensuring optimal management of GERD and reducing the risk of Barrett's Esophagus.

How to Assess Personal Risk Factors

Assessing personal risk factors for Barrett's Esophagus involves a comprehensive evaluation of lifestyle, health history, and symptoms. Individuals can start by reflecting on their eating habits, physical activity levels, and any existing health conditions. This self-assessment can provide valuable insights into potential risks and necessary lifestyle adjustments.

Consulting with healthcare professionals is essential for a thorough risk assessment. Medical evaluations may include discussions about family history, existing GERD symptoms, and lifestyle choices. This collaborative approach enables individuals to develop tailored prevention strategies based on their unique risk profiles.

Importance of Lifestyle Changes to Mitigate Risks

Lifestyle changes are critical in reducing the risk of Barrett's Esophagus and managing GERD symptoms. Incorporating regular physical activity, maintaining a healthy weight, and avoiding known irritants, such as tobacco and excessive alcohol, can significantly improve esophageal health. These changes not only alleviate symptoms but also enhance overall well-being.

To implement effective lifestyle changes, individuals can start by setting realistic goals and gradually incorporating healthier habits into their daily routines. Engaging in activities such as cooking nutritious meals, participating in regular exercise, and practicing stress management techniques can contribute to long-term health improvements and a reduced risk of Barrett's Esophagus.

Recommendations for Screening Based on Risk

Screening for Barrett's Esophagus is particularly important for individuals at higher risk, such as those with long-standing GERD or a family history of esophageal cancer. Healthcare providers may recommend endoscopy as a screening tool to detect any abnormal changes in the esophagus early. Understanding when and how to seek screening can help in early intervention.

Individuals should discuss their personal risk factors with their healthcare providers to determine the appropriate screening schedule. Regular follow-ups and adherence to screening recommendations can ensure early detection and management of Barrett's Esophagus, ultimately improving health outcomes.

Future Research Directions on Causes and Prevention

Future research on Barrett's Esophagus focuses on understanding the underlying causes and developing effective prevention strategies. This includes exploring genetic factors, dietary influences, and environmental exposures that contribute to the condition. Advancements in research can lead to more personalized approaches to managing and preventing Barrett's Esophagus.

Staying informed about ongoing research can empower individuals to adopt evidence-based practices in their health management. Participating in clinical studies or following emerging guidelines can enhance understanding and contribute to the collective effort in addressing Barrett's Esophagus effectively.

CHAPTER 3:

Dietary Changes for Management

Importance of Diet in Managing Barrett's Esophagus

Diet plays a crucial role in managing Barrett's Esophagus, primarily due to its association with gastroesophageal reflux disease (GERD). By adopting a balanced diet, patients can reduce inflammation, lower acid production, and alleviate symptoms like heartburn and discomfort. Focusing on dietary changes can help improve esophageal health and may even reduce the risk of progression to esophageal cancer.

To manage Barrett's Esophagus effectively, individuals should prioritize anti-inflammatory foods while limiting those that trigger reflux symptoms. This means incorporating fruits, vegetables, whole grains, and lean proteins while avoiding high-fat and spicy foods. With careful dietary planning, patients can better control their symptoms and enhance their overall quality of life.

Foods to Include for Better Esophageal Health

Including a variety of nutrient-dense foods can promote better esophageal health for those with Barrett's Esophagus. Foods rich in antioxidants, such as berries, leafy greens, and nuts, can help reduce inflammation and support overall digestive health. Additionally, whole grains like oatmeal and brown rice can aid digestion and keep acid levels in check.

Incorporating healthy fats, such as avocados and olive oil, can also be beneficial. These fats help soothe the esophagus and reduce irritation. Aim to build meals around these foods to create a balanced diet that supports your digestive system while minimizing the risk of symptoms.

Foods to Avoid to Minimize Symptoms

To minimize symptoms associated with Barrett's Esophagus, certain foods should be avoided. Spicy foods, citrus fruits, and tomatoes can exacerbate heartburn and irritation, so it's best to limit or eliminate these items from your diet. Additionally, high-fat foods, including fried items and full-fat dairy, can increase acid production, leading to discomfort.

Caffeinated beverages, carbonated drinks, and alcohol can also trigger reflux symptoms. Being mindful of these foods and drinks will help in managing Barrett's Esophagus symptoms effectively, allowing for a more comfortable dining experience.

Suggested Meal Planning Tips for Barrett's Esophagus

Meal planning is essential for individuals with Barrett's Esophagus to ensure they stay on track with their dietary goals. Start by creating a weekly menu that features a variety of allowed foods, focusing on colorful fruits and vegetables, whole grains, and lean proteins. Prepare meals in advance to avoid last-minute unhealthy choices and help you stay consistent.

Incorporating snacks throughout the day can help maintain energy levels and prevent overeating at meal times. Keep healthy snacks, such as cut vegetables, nuts, or yogurt, readily available to promote better eating habits while minimizing reflux triggers.

The Role of Fiber in Digestive Health

Fiber is an important component of a healthy diet, especially for those with Barrett's Esophagus. It aids digestion, promotes regular bowel movements, and helps maintain a healthy weight, all of which are vital for managing symptoms. Incorporating high-fiber foods, such as fruits, vegetables, legumes, and whole grains, can support digestive health and reduce the likelihood of reflux.

To increase fiber intake, consider starting your day with a high-fiber breakfast, such as oatmeal topped with fruit or a smoothie with leafy greens and berries. Gradually adding fiber-rich foods to your meals will help your body adjust, minimizing any digestive discomfort while providing essential nutrients.

How to Read Food Labels Effectively

Understanding food labels is essential for making informed choices when managing Barrett's Esophagus. Start by looking at the serving size, as this can significantly impact calorie and nutrient content. Next, pay attention to the total fat and sugar content; aim for foods lower in saturated fats and added sugars to promote better health.

Additionally, check for specific ingredients that may trigger symptoms, such as high-fat content, caffeine, or spicy seasonings. Familiarizing yourself with common food additives and their effects will empower you to make healthier decisions when shopping, ensuring your diet supports esophageal health.

Importance of Hydration for Esophageal Health

Staying hydrated is vital for overall health, including esophageal function. Drinking plenty of water helps to dilute stomach acids and flush out irritants from the digestive system. Aim for at least 8 cups of water daily, adjusting based on your activity level and individual needs to support optimal hydration.

Incorporating hydrating foods, such as cucumbers, watermelon, and soups, can also enhance your fluid intake. Avoid overly acidic beverages, like citrus juices or sodas, which can aggravate the esophagus, opting instead for water or herbal teas to stay hydrated and soothe irritation.

Benefits of Smaller, More Frequent Meals

Eating smaller, more frequent meals can help manage symptoms of Barrett's Esophagus effectively. Instead of three large meals, aim for five to six smaller meals throughout the day to prevent excessive pressure on the stomach and reduce the likelihood of reflux. This approach can also help maintain steady energy levels and support better digestion.

To implement this strategy, plan your meals and snacks in advance, ensuring they are balanced and include a variety of foods. Keeping portions moderate can prevent overeating, allowing you to enjoy your food without triggering uncomfortable symptoms.

Suggestions for Cooking Methods to Reduce Irritation

Choosing the right cooking methods can make a significant difference in managing Barrett's Esophagus. Opt for methods like steaming, baking, or grilling instead of frying or sautéing in oil, as these healthier techniques can help preserve nutrients while minimizing added fats that can exacerbate symptoms.

When cooking, focus on using herbs and spices that are gentle on the stomach, such as basil or parsley, rather than hot spices. Experiment with various cooking styles to find the best options that suit your taste while ensuring a comforting and nutritious meal.

Nutritional Supplements That May Help

Certain nutritional supplements may support esophageal health for those with Barrett's Esophagus. Probiotics, for example, can help maintain a healthy gut microbiome and improve digestion. Omega-3 fatty acids, found in fish oil or flaxseed oil, can also help reduce inflammation throughout the body.

Before starting any supplement, consult with a healthcare provider to ensure they are appropriate for your specific needs and to determine the correct dosages. Combining supplements with a balanced diet can optimize your health and enhance the management of Barrett's Esophagus.

Importance of Keeping a Food Diary

Keeping a food diary can be a valuable tool for managing Barrett's Esophagus symptoms. By tracking what you eat and noting any symptoms experienced afterward, you can identify specific foods or habits that may trigger reflux or discomfort. This self-awareness will empower you to make better dietary choices.

To start a food diary, write down everything you eat and drink, along with the times and any symptoms you experience. Review your entries regularly to spot patterns and adjust your diet accordingly, making informed decisions that support your esophageal health.

Strategies for Dining Out Safely

Dining out can pose challenges for those managing Barrett's Esophagus, but with some strategies, it can be enjoyable. Start by researching restaurant menus in advance to identify suitable options and communicate your dietary needs to the staff. Consider calling ahead to inquire about how meals are prepared and to request modifications.

When at the restaurant, opt for dishes that are grilled, steamed, or baked rather than fried, and ask for dressings and sauces on the side. By being proactive and mindful of your choices, you can enjoy dining out while minimizing the risk of symptoms.

Adjusting Recipes to Suit Dietary Needs

Adapting recipes to suit your dietary needs for Barrett's Esophagus is both practical and rewarding. Start by identifying recipes that contain trigger ingredients and brainstorm substitutions. For example, replace acidic ingredients like tomatoes with milder options such as pumpkin or squash to reduce irritation.

Experimenting with cooking techniques and flavoring methods can also enhance your meals. Use herbs, spices, and gentle cooking methods to create dishes that are flavorful yet easy on your esophagus, ensuring you maintain a nutritious and enjoyable diet.

CHAPTER 4:

Support Strategies for Living with Barrett's Esophagus

Importance of a Support Network (Friends, Family, Support Groups)

A robust support network is essential for individuals managing Barrett's esophagus. Friends and family can offer emotional backing, practical assistance, and a sense of belonging, making it easier to navigate the challenges of the condition. Engaging with support groups—whether in-person or online—can provide valuable insights and shared experiences from others facing similar health issues. This community aspect fosters understanding and reduces feelings of isolation, making it crucial for mental well-being.

To effectively build your support network, start by reaching out to those closest to you. Communicate your needs and experiences to family and friends, encouraging them to participate in discussions about your health. Look for local or virtual support groups specific to Barrett's esophagus or GERD where you can connect with others. Websites and social media platforms can help you find groups, allowing for a more extensive exchange of experiences and tips on managing symptoms and making lifestyle adjustments.

Psychological Support: Counseling and Stress Management

Psychological support plays a vital role in managing Barrett's esophagus. Counseling can help patients cope with anxiety, depression, and stress associated with their condition. A professional therapist can provide strategies to manage negative emotions, improving overall mental health and resilience. Techniques like cognitive-behavioral therapy (CBT) can be particularly effective in helping individuals reframe their thoughts and reactions to stressors.

In addition to counseling, stress management techniques such as mindfulness, meditation, and relaxation exercises can significantly benefit those dealing with Barrett's esophagus. Setting aside time each day for deep breathing or guided meditation can enhance emotional stability. Many free resources are available online, including apps and videos, to help you integrate these practices into your daily routine.

Education Resources for Patients and Families

Education is a cornerstone of effective Barrett's esophagus management. Understanding the condition, its causes, and its implications empowers patients and families to make informed decisions. Reliable resources, such as patient advocacy organizations and medical websites, provide comprehensive information on Barrett's esophagus, including dietary changes and lifestyle modifications.

Families should also engage in educational sessions with healthcare providers. This collaboration can clarify treatment options and create a tailored management plan. Make use of pamphlets, online courses, and webinars that focus on Barrett's esophagus and GERD. These resources can be invaluable for staying updated on the latest research and recommended practices.

Working with Healthcare Providers for Optimal Care

Collaboration with healthcare providers is essential for managing Barrett's esophagus effectively. Regular check-ups and discussions about your symptoms can ensure timely adjustments to your treatment plan. Make a habit of preparing for appointments by writing down your questions and concerns, so you leave with a clear understanding of your care strategy.

It's also important to establish a relationship based on trust and open communication with your healthcare team. Discuss any changes in your symptoms or side effects of medications promptly. This proactive approach allows for better management of the condition and can lead to improved health outcomes over time.

Importance of Communicating Symptoms and Concerns

Effective communication about symptoms and concerns is crucial in managing Barrett's esophagus. Keeping a symptom diary can help track what triggers your symptoms, making it easier to discuss this information with your healthcare provider. Note the frequency, intensity, and duration of symptoms to identify patterns and potential food triggers.

Don't hesitate to express any concerns regarding treatment or lifestyle changes during your healthcare visits. Clear communication can lead to adjustments in your care plan that better fit your lifestyle and health needs. This openness encourages a collaborative approach to managing your condition, ensuring you feel supported and informed throughout your journey.

Techniques for Managing Anxiety Related to Health

Managing anxiety related to Barrett's esophagus can significantly enhance your quality of life. Techniques such as deep breathing exercises, progressive muscle relaxation, and mindfulness meditation can be effective in reducing anxiety symptoms. Regular practice of these methods can help calm your mind and allow you to approach your health concerns more positively.

Additionally, engaging in hobbies or activities that bring you joy can serve as effective distractions from anxiety. Establish a routine that incorporates physical activity, such as walking or yoga, which is known to reduce stress levels. Finding a balance between self-care and health management can create a more positive mindset, helping you cope with anxiety.

How to Set Realistic Health Goals

Setting realistic health goals is vital for managing Barrett's esophagus. Start by identifying specific, measurable, achievable, relevant, and time-bound (SMART) goals related to your health. For instance, aim to incorporate a specific number of fruits and vegetables into your daily diet or to engage in physical activity for a set amount of time each week.

Break these goals down into smaller, manageable steps to avoid feeling overwhelmed. Celebrate small victories along the way to maintain motivation. Regularly reassess your goals, adjusting them as needed to reflect changes in your health or lifestyle, ensuring they remain relevant and achievable.

The Role of Physical Activity in Overall Well-Being

Physical activity is crucial for enhancing overall well-being, particularly for those with Barrett's esophagus. Regular exercise can help manage weight, improve digestion, and reduce the severity of GERD symptoms. Aim for a balanced routine that includes aerobic exercises, strength training, and flexibility activities to support your health.

Incorporating physical activity into your daily routine doesn't have to be overwhelming. Start with small changes, such as taking short walks or choosing stairs over elevators. Gradually increase your activity level, aiming for at least 150 minutes of moderate-intensity exercise each week. Listen to your body and adjust your routine based on how you feel.

Tips for Coping with Lifestyle Changes

Coping with lifestyle changes due to Barrett's esophagus can be challenging but manageable with the right strategies. Begin by identifying specific changes you need to make, such as dietary adjustments or the elimination of certain foods. Gradually implement these changes to avoid feeling deprived, allowing yourself time to adapt.

Involve family and friends in your lifestyle changes to create a supportive environment. Share your goals and encourage them to participate in healthy activities together. By fostering a collaborative atmosphere, you can make the transition smoother and more enjoyable, reinforcing positive habits.

Encouragement to Share Experiences with Others

Sharing experiences with others who have Barrett's esophagus can be incredibly beneficial. Open discussions can provide emotional relief, valuable insights, and practical tips for managing symptoms. Consider joining support groups, either locally or online, where you can connect with others who understand your journey.

Be open about your experiences in these settings, as it can help build a sense of community and mutual support. Engaging in conversations about challenges and triumphs fosters an environment of understanding, reducing feelings of isolation and encouraging shared learning.

Utilizing Online Resources and Forums for Support

Online resources and forums can be valuable tools for managing Barrett's esophagus. Websites dedicated to gastrointestinal health provide articles, research, and forums where individuals can ask questions and share experiences. These platforms can help you stay informed about new treatments, dietary recommendations, and lifestyle tips.

Participating in online forums allows you to connect with others facing similar challenges. Share your insights, ask for advice, and learn from the experiences of others. These interactions can enrich your understanding of the condition and provide a supportive community, helping you feel less alone in your journey.

Importance of Self-Advocacy in Healthcare

Self-advocacy is essential in managing Barrett's esophagus. Taking an active role in your healthcare means understanding your condition, treatment options, and rights as a patient. Educate yourself about Barrett's esophagus through reputable sources, enabling you to ask informed questions and make empowered decisions regarding your health.

Being assertive during healthcare appointments is crucial. Don't hesitate to voice concerns, request clarification on treatment plans, and express your preferences regarding your care. By advocating for yourself, you help ensure that your needs are met, fostering a more collaborative relationship with your healthcare providers.

Resources for Local Support Groups and Organizations

Finding local support groups and organizations dedicated to Barrett's esophagus can provide a wealth of resources and community support. Start by checking with local hospitals, healthcare facilities, or patient advocacy organizations for information on available groups. Many communities host meetings where patients can share experiences and gain support from others facing similar challenges.

In addition to in-person groups, consider exploring online directories that list support organizations. Websites such as the American Gastroenterological Association or the International Foundation for Gastrointestinal Disorders offer tools to connect you with local resources. Participating in these groups can enhance your support network and provide valuable insights into managing Barrett's esophagus effectively.

CHAPTER 5:

Early Intervention and Regular Monitoring

Importance of Regular Check-Ups with Healthcare Providers

Regular check-ups with healthcare providers are crucial for individuals diagnosed with Barrett's Esophagus, as they help monitor changes in the condition and prevent complications. During these appointments, your healthcare team can evaluate your symptoms, conduct necessary tests, and adjust treatment plans accordingly. Being proactive about your health ensures any potential issues are addressed promptly, allowing for better management of your condition.

To make the most of these visits, prepare a list of any new symptoms or concerns you may have experienced since your last appointment. This will help your doctor understand your situation more comprehensively and tailor recommendations or treatments specifically to your needs.

Recommended Frequency for Monitoring Barrett's Esophagus

The recommended frequency for monitoring Barrett's Esophagus typically depends on the severity of the condition and individual risk factors. Generally, patients may be advised to undergo surveillance endoscopies every three to five years; however, those with higher risk factors for progression to esophageal cancer may require more frequent evaluations.

To establish a personalized monitoring schedule, discuss your specific risk factors and health status with your healthcare provider. Staying informed about your monitoring plan allows you to be proactive in managing your health and detecting any changes early.

Understanding the Role of Biopsies and Pathology Reports

Biopsies are a crucial part of diagnosing Barrett's Esophagus and determining the presence of dysplasia, which can indicate a risk of cancer. During an endoscopy, small samples of the esophageal lining are taken and sent to a laboratory for analysis. The pathology report generated will detail the findings, helping your healthcare provider devise an appropriate treatment plan.

Understanding your pathology report is vital. Take the time to review it with your doctor, asking questions about the implications of the results and how they affect your overall management plan. This knowledge empowers you to make informed decisions about your treatment options.

Importance of Esophageal Cancer Awareness

Awareness of esophageal cancer is essential for individuals with Barrett's Esophagus, as it can increase your understanding of potential risks and symptoms to watch for. Being aware of risk factors such as chronic gastroesophageal reflux disease (GERD), obesity, and smoking can help you take proactive measures to mitigate those risks.

Regular education about esophageal cancer symptoms, such as difficulty swallowing or unintentional weight loss, can also enhance early detection. By understanding these risks and symptoms, you can work closely with your healthcare provider to monitor your health and act swiftly if any concerning changes arise.

How to Recognize Changes in Symptoms

Recognizing changes in symptoms is vital for managing Barrett's Esophagus effectively. Common symptoms to monitor include persistent heartburn, regurgitation of food or sour liquid, chest pain, and difficulty swallowing. Keeping a symptom diary can help you track when symptoms occur and their intensity, which can provide valuable insights during medical appointments.

If you notice any new or worsening symptoms, it's essential to report them to your healthcare provider promptly. Early recognition and reporting can lead to timely interventions, helping to prevent complications and ensure your treatment remains effective.

Benefits of Early Treatment Interventions

Early treatment interventions can significantly impact the management of Barrett's Esophagus and reduce the risk of progression to esophageal cancer. Treatments may include lifestyle changes, medication, or more invasive procedures, depending on the severity of the condition. Initiating these treatments promptly can improve symptoms and help prevent further complications.

To implement early interventions, work with your healthcare provider to establish a tailored treatment plan that addresses your specific needs. Adopting dietary changes, using medications like proton pump inhibitors (PPIs), or considering endoscopic therapies can all be effective strategies when initiated early.

The Role of Proton Pump Inhibitors (PPIs) and Other Medications

Proton pump inhibitors (PPIs) play a vital role in managing Barrett's Esophagus by reducing stomach acid production, which helps alleviate symptoms and prevent damage to the esophagus. Commonly prescribed PPIs include omeprazole and lansoprazole. It's important to take these medications as directed by your healthcare provider for optimal results.

In addition to PPIs, other medications may be prescribed based on individual needs. Always communicate with your healthcare provider about your treatment plan and any concerns you may have regarding medications. Understanding how these drugs work can enhance adherence and empower you in managing your condition.

Understanding Your Treatment Options

Understanding your treatment options for Barrett's Esophagus is essential for making informed decisions about your care. Treatments can range from lifestyle modifications and medications to more invasive procedures like endoscopic mucosal resection or radiofrequency ablation. Each option has its indications and potential benefits, so discussing these thoroughly with your healthcare provider is crucial.

To navigate these options effectively, ask questions about the risks, benefits, and expected outcomes of each treatment. Being well-informed allows you to actively participate in discussions about your care and make choices that align with your health goals.

Importance of Follow-Up Appointments After Diagnosis

Follow-up appointments are crucial after a Barrett's Esophagus diagnosis, as they allow for ongoing monitoring and adjustments to your treatment plan. During these visits, your healthcare provider can assess how well you're managing symptoms, review any test results, and determine if further action is needed. Regular follow-ups help ensure that any changes in your condition are addressed promptly.

To maximize the benefit of follow-up visits, maintain an updated list of questions or concerns related to your health. This proactive approach encourages open communication with your healthcare provider and helps ensure you receive the most appropriate care based on your current situation.

Keeping an Organized Health Record

Keeping an organized health record is essential for effective management of Barrett's Esophagus. This record should include medical history, medications, symptoms, and results from tests and procedures. An organized health record helps you track your condition over time and provides valuable information during medical appointments.

To create a comprehensive health record, consider using a digital tool or a simple notebook to log information consistently. This practice not only empowers you to take an active role in your health care but also improves communication with your healthcare team.

Utilizing Technology for Health Tracking

Utilizing technology for health tracking can significantly enhance your ability to manage

Barrett's Esophagus. Various apps and wearable devices allow you to monitor symptoms, track medication adherence, and even log dietary habits. These tools can provide valuable insights and help identify triggers that may worsen your condition.

To get started, explore available health tracking apps or devices that align with your preferences and needs. Regularly reviewing the data you collect can help you and your healthcare provider make informed decisions about your treatment and lifestyle changes.

Importance of Adhering to Medical Advice

Adhering to medical advice is crucial for effectively managing Barrett's Esophagus and preventing complications. This includes following prescribed treatment plans, attending regular check-ups, and implementing lifestyle changes recommended by your healthcare provider. Consistent adherence can lead to improved outcomes and a better quality of life.

To ensure adherence, consider setting reminders for medications and appointments, and actively engage in discussions about your treatment plan. Understanding the rationale behind medical advice can also motivate you to follow recommendations more closely, fostering a collaborative relationship with your healthcare team.

CHAPTER 6:

Lifestyle Modifications for Better Health

Overview of Lifestyle Changes That Support Esophageal Health

Making lifestyle changes is crucial for supporting esophageal health, particularly for individuals with Barrett's Esophagus. Key adjustments include adopting a balanced diet rich in fruits, vegetables, and whole grains while reducing intake of processed foods, spicy dishes, and high-fat items. These changes can help minimize acid reflux and promote better digestive health.

Incorporating smaller, more frequent meals instead of larger ones can also reduce pressure on the esophagus. Keeping a food diary to track what triggers symptoms can be beneficial for identifying problematic foods and habits. Regularly discussing these changes with a healthcare professional can provide additional guidance tailored to individual needs.

Importance of Weight Management

Maintaining a healthy weight is essential for managing Barrett's Esophagus, as excess weight can increase abdominal pressure and contribute to acid reflux. Simple strategies to achieve weight management include incorporating physical activity into daily routines, such as walking, cycling, or swimming. Aim for at least 150 minutes of moderate exercise each week to support weight loss and overall health.

In addition to physical activity, focusing on portion control and mindful eating can aid in weight management. Using smaller plates, paying attention to hunger cues, and avoiding distractions while eating can help prevent overeating. Working with a registered dietitian can provide personalized meal planning to meet weight loss goals.

Smoking Cessation Strategies and Resources

Quitting smoking is vital for improving esophageal health and reducing the risk of Barrett's Esophagus progression. Several effective strategies include setting a quit date, identifying triggers, and finding alternative coping mechanisms. Using resources such as quitlines, mobile apps, or support groups can provide the necessary encouragement and accountability.

Nicotine replacement therapies (NRTs) like patches or gum can help ease withdrawal symptoms. Additionally, exploring mindfulness techniques or behavioral therapies can further support quitting efforts. Seeking guidance from healthcare providers can enhance success rates and develop a personalized cessation plan.

Impact of Alcohol Consumption on Barrett's Esophagus

Alcohol consumption can exacerbate symptoms of Barrett's Esophagus by relaxing the lower esophageal sphincter and increasing acid reflux. To manage this condition effectively, individuals should limit or eliminate alcohol intake. Start by gradually reducing consumption, perhaps through designated alcohol-free days or choosing lower-alcohol beverages.

Consider discussing alcohol's impact on health with a healthcare professional to gain insight into personal limits. Joining support groups focused on alcohol moderation can provide additional motivation and resources for those seeking to make significant lifestyle changes.

Strategies for Improving Sleep Quality

Quality sleep is crucial for overall health and can impact esophageal symptoms. To improve sleep quality, create a consistent sleep schedule by going to bed and waking up at the same time daily. Establish a relaxing bedtime routine that includes activities such as reading, gentle stretching, or deep breathing exercises to signal your body that it's time to wind down.

Additionally, consider adjusting the sleep environment by keeping the bedroom dark, cool, and quiet. Elevating the head of the bed can help minimize nighttime reflux symptoms. If sleep issues persist, consulting a healthcare professional for evaluation and personalized recommendations can be beneficial.

The Importance of Stress Reduction Techniques

Managing stress is essential for individuals with Barrett's Esophagus, as stress can worsen symptoms and trigger reflux. Implementing stress reduction techniques such as deep breathing exercises, meditation, or yoga can promote relaxation. Setting aside time each day for mindfulness practices can help cultivate a sense of calm.

Engaging in enjoyable activities, such as hobbies or spending time with loved ones, can also reduce stress levels. Consider keeping a journal to reflect on daily experiences and feelings, which can provide insights into stress triggers and coping strategies. Working with a therapist can offer additional support in managing stress effectively.

Physical Activities That Are Safe and Beneficial

Incorporating safe physical activities into daily life can enhance overall health and support esophageal well-being. Low-impact exercises such as walking, swimming, or cycling are beneficial and easy to integrate into most routines. Aim for at least 30 minutes of physical activity most days of the week to promote cardiovascular health and maintain a healthy weight.

It's important to listen to your body and avoid high-impact activities that could exacerbate symptoms. Start slowly and gradually increase the intensity and duration of workouts. Seeking guidance from a healthcare provider or physical therapist can help develop a safe exercise plan tailored to individual needs.

Techniques for Mindfulness and Relaxation

Mindfulness and relaxation techniques can significantly benefit those with Barrett's Esophagus by reducing stress and promoting emotional well-being. Practices such as guided meditation, progressive muscle relaxation, or mindfulness-based stress reduction can enhance awareness of physical sensations and emotional responses.

Setting aside a few minutes daily for these practices can create a calming routine that helps manage symptoms. Utilizing apps or online resources can make learning these techniques more accessible. Consider joining a local class or group to foster connection and support while practicing mindfulness.

Importance of Routine Health Screenings

Routine health screenings play a crucial role in monitoring Barrett's Esophagus and preventing complications. Regular check-ups with a healthcare provider can help identify any changes in symptoms and allow for timely interventions. It's important to follow recommended screening guidelines, which may include endoscopies to assess the esophagus's condition.

Keeping an organized record of medical appointments, screenings, and results can facilitate effective communication with healthcare providers. Establishing a proactive approach to health management can significantly impact long-term outcomes and overall well-being.

Building a Healthy Living Environment

Creating a healthy living environment is vital for managing Barrett's Esophagus. Start by decluttering your home and minimizing exposure to allergens or irritants, such as smoke or strong odors. Designating areas for relaxation and stress relief, such as a reading nook or garden, can contribute to a calming atmosphere.

Incorporating healthy food options within easy reach can also encourage better dietary choices. Consider engaging family members in discussions about healthy living to foster a supportive environment. Establishing routines that promote well-being can create a nurturing space for everyone.

Community Resources for Lifestyle Changes

Accessing community resources can significantly enhance efforts to implement lifestyle changes for Barrett's Esophagus. Local health organizations, support groups, and wellness programs often provide valuable information and support. Participating in community workshops or seminars can deepen understanding of effective lifestyle modifications.

Online forums and social media groups can also connect individuals facing similar challenges, providing an avenue for sharing experiences and tips. Utilize local libraries or community centers for resources and programs focused on health education and lifestyle improvement.

Engaging in Hobbies That Promote Well-Being

Engaging in hobbies can significantly improve overall well-being and provide a positive distraction from symptoms of Barrett's Esophagus. Consider exploring activities such as gardening, painting, or crafting, which can foster creativity and relaxation. Finding a hobby that brings joy can enhance mood and decrease stress levels.

Scheduling regular time for these activities can encourage consistency and promote mental health. Joining clubs or classes can also facilitate social connections while engaging in enjoyable pastimes, contributing to a well-rounded lifestyle.

Encouragement for Sustainable Lifestyle Choices

Encouraging sustainable lifestyle choices is essential for long-term management of Barrett's Esophagus.

Aim to make gradual changes rather than overwhelming yourself with drastic shifts. Focus on adopting habits that align with personal values and goals, promoting a sense of agency in the process.

Consider setting realistic, achievable goals, such as incorporating more fruits and vegetables into meals or gradually increasing physical activity. Celebrating small successes along the way can foster motivation and commitment to maintaining healthier lifestyle choices over time.

CHAPTER 7:

Understanding Treatments and Medications

Overview of Medical Treatments for Barrett's Esophagus

Barrett's Esophagus is often treated through a combination of lifestyle changes, medications, and surgical interventions. Common medical treatments include proton pump inhibitors (PPIs) to reduce stomach acid production, endoscopic procedures like radiofrequency ablation, and surveillance through regular endoscopies. Patients should consult with their healthcare provider to determine the most appropriate treatment plan based on the severity of their condition.

In addition to medications, some patients may benefit from surgical options such as fundoplication, where the top of the stomach is wrapped around the lower esophagus to prevent acid reflux. Regular follow-up visits are crucial to monitor the progression of Barrett's Esophagus and adjust treatments as needed.

Importance of Discussing Medication Options with a Doctor

Open communication with a healthcare provider is vital for managing Barrett's Esophagus effectively. Patients should discuss their symptoms, medical history, and any concerns regarding potential medications. This collaborative approach allows for a tailored treatment plan that addresses individual needs and preferences.

When discussing medication options, it's essential to ask about the expected benefits, duration of treatment, and possible side effects. This proactive dialogue helps patients make informed decisions and ensures they are comfortable with their prescribed treatments.

Side Effects and Benefits of Common Medications (e.g., PPIs)

Proton pump inhibitors (PPIs) are commonly prescribed to manage Barrett's Esophagus by controlling acid production. While effective in reducing symptoms of gastroesophageal reflux disease (GERD) and preventing further damage to the esophagus, PPIs can have side effects such as headaches, gastrointestinal disturbances, and long-term risks like nutrient deficiencies and kidney disease.

Patients should weigh the benefits of symptom relief and potential esophageal healing against the risks of long-term medication use. Regular check-ins with healthcare providers can help in assessing the medication's effectiveness and managing any side effects that may arise.

Alternative Therapies and Their Role in Treatment

Alternative therapies can complement traditional medical treatments for Barrett's Esophagus. Options such as dietary changes, herbal supplements, and acupuncture may help alleviate symptoms and improve overall well-being. A diet rich in fruits, vegetables, and whole grains can help reduce inflammation and promote digestive health.

Before starting any alternative therapy, it is crucial to consult with a healthcare provider to ensure these methods are safe and appropriate for individual health conditions. Integrating alternative therapies with standard treatments can enhance patient outcomes and provide additional support.

The Role of Surgical Interventions When Necessary

Surgical interventions may become necessary for patients with Barrett's Esophagus who do not respond well to medical treatment or who develop high-grade dysplasia. Procedures like endoscopic mucosal resection (EMR) and esophagectomy (removal of part or all of the esophagus) aim to eliminate cancerous cells and reduce the risk of progression to esophageal cancer.

Patients should discuss the potential benefits and risks of surgical options with their healthcare team. Understanding what to expect during recovery and follow-up care is essential for a successful outcome.

Importance of Personalized Treatment Plans

Every patient with Barrett's Esophagus is unique, necessitating a personalized treatment plan that takes into account individual symptoms, health history, and lifestyle factors. This tailored approach enhances the effectiveness of treatment and improves patient adherence to the recommended plan.

Working closely with healthcare providers allows for adjustments in treatment as the patient's condition evolves. A personalized plan may involve a combination of medications, lifestyle modifications, and monitoring to achieve the best possible results.

Monitoring Effectiveness of Prescribed Treatments

Regular monitoring of the effectiveness of prescribed treatments is crucial in managing Barrett's Esophagus. Patients should schedule follow-up appointments to evaluate their response to medications, review symptom improvement, and undergo necessary endoscopies to assess changes in the esophagus.

Keeping a symptom diary can be a helpful tool for patients to track changes over time, enabling them to share this information with their healthcare provider. This collaborative approach facilitates timely adjustments to treatment as needed.

Communicating with Healthcare Providers About Medications

Effective communication with healthcare providers about medications is essential for optimal management of Barrett's Esophagus. Patients should openly discuss any side effects experienced, concerns about drug interactions, and questions regarding their treatment plan.

Engaging in this dialogue helps ensure that the prescribed medications are the best fit for the patient's needs. Being proactive about communication fosters a strong patient-provider relationship and encourages better health outcomes.

Understanding Drug Interactions and Contraindications

Patients should be aware of potential drug interactions and contraindications when taking medications for Barrett's Esophagus. Certain medications may interfere with the effectiveness of PPIs or other treatments, leading to decreased symptom control.

Discussing all medications, including over-the-counter drugs and supplements, with healthcare providers is critical to preventing adverse effects. This comprehensive approach helps create a safer and more effective treatment regimen.

Keeping Track of Medication Schedules

Maintaining a consistent medication schedule is vital for the effective management of Barrett's Esophagus. Patients can use pill organizers, mobile apps, or reminders to ensure they take their medications as prescribed.

Staying organized not only helps avoid missed doses but also reinforces the importance of adherence to the treatment plan. Consistency in medication intake plays a significant role in symptom control and overall health.

Research on New Treatment Options

Staying informed about research on new treatment options for Barrett's Esophagus is essential for patients seeking the latest advancements in care. Clinical trials often explore innovative therapies and medications that may offer additional benefits beyond standard treatments.

Patients interested in participating in clinical trials should discuss this with their healthcare provider, who can provide guidance on eligibility and potential risks. Engaging in research can lead to new treatment opportunities and contribute to advancements in Barrett's Esophagus management.

Importance of Clinical Trials and Research Participation

Participating in clinical trials is crucial for the advancement of treatment options for Barrett's Esophagus. These studies allow patients to access cutting-edge therapies and contribute to the body of knowledge that shapes future care.

Patients should consider the potential benefits and risks of participating in a clinical trial. Discussing these options with healthcare providers can help determine if a trial is appropriate for their condition and treatment goals.

Patient Stories and Experiences with Treatment

Listening to patient stories and experiences can provide valuable insights into managing Barrett's

Esophagus. Hearing about others' journeys can offer hope, practical tips, and encouragement during challenging times.

Sharing experiences through support groups or online communities can foster connection and understanding. This exchange of information helps patients feel less isolated and empowers them to take an active role in their treatment journey.

CHAPTER 8:

Complications and Emergency Situations

Overview of Potential Complications Associated with Barrett's Esophagus

Barrett's esophagus can lead to various complications, primarily due to the changes in the esophageal lining. The most significant concern is the increased risk of esophageal adenocarcinoma, a type of cancer that can develop from the precancerous cells in the Barrett's tissue. Other complications may include strictures or narrowing of the esophagus, leading to swallowing difficulties and chronic inflammation.

To manage these complications effectively, regular surveillance through endoscopy is crucial. This allows for early detection and intervention, reducing the risk of progression to cancer. Patients should stay informed about their condition and discuss any changes in symptoms with their healthcare provider, ensuring timely action when necessary.

Understanding the Risk of Esophageal Cancer

Patients with Barrett's esophagus are at a higher risk for developing esophageal cancer, specifically esophageal adenocarcinoma. This risk increases with the duration of Barrett's esophagus and the degree of dysplasia observed in biopsies. Dysplasia refers to abnormal cells that have the potential to become cancerous over time. Therefore, regular monitoring and endoscopic evaluations are essential for those diagnosed with Barrett's.

To mitigate cancer risk, patients should adopt lifestyle changes such as quitting smoking, reducing alcohol consumption, and maintaining a healthy weight. Additionally, discussing personalized surveillance schedules with healthcare providers helps ensure that any potential progression towards cancer is caught early, allowing for timely intervention.

Signs of Complications That Require Immediate Attention

Certain signs may indicate complications from Barrett's esophagus that necessitate immediate medical attention. These include difficulty swallowing (dysphagia), persistent chest pain, unexplained weight loss, or vomiting blood. Such symptoms may signal the development of strictures or even malignancy, and prompt evaluation is vital.

When experiencing these alarming symptoms, it's important to contact your healthcare provider immediately or seek emergency care. Early recognition and treatment of these complications can significantly improve outcomes and reduce the risk of severe health issues.

The Importance of Emergency Care and When to Seek It

Emergency care is essential for managing severe complications associated with Barrett's esophagus. Conditions like significant bleeding, acute chest pain, or sudden difficulty in swallowing should prompt immediate medical evaluation. Understanding when to seek emergency care can be lifesaving and prevent further complications.

In an emergency, it is helpful to have a list of your symptoms, medications, and medical history ready for the healthcare provider. This information aids in quicker diagnosis and treatment, ensuring that any urgent issues are addressed without delay.

Strategies for Managing Acute Symptoms

Managing acute symptoms of Barrett's esophagus often involves a combination of medication and lifestyle adjustments. Over-the-counter antacids, H2 blockers, or proton pump inhibitors (PPIs) can provide relief from heartburn and acid reflux. Additionally, avoiding trigger foods—such as spicy, acidic, or fatty foods—can help minimize symptoms.

Creating a food diary may help identify and avoid personal triggers more effectively. Regular meals, rather than large portions, can also reduce the likelihood of acute symptoms, allowing for better management of the condition.

Understanding the Role of Advanced Diagnostic Tools

Advanced diagnostic tools, such as endoscopy and biopsy, play a crucial role in managing Barrett's esophagus. These procedures allow doctors to visualize the esophagus and assess the extent of Barrett's changes. Biopsy samples can determine the presence of dysplasia, guiding further treatment options.

Regular screening through these advanced tools is vital for early detection of potential complications. Patients should discuss with their healthcare providers how often these tests should be performed based on their individual risk factors and history.

Importance of Patient Education on Complications

Patient education is key to effectively managing Barrett's esophagus and its potential complications. Understanding the disease, its risks, and possible symptoms empowers patients to take an active role in their healthcare. Educational resources, such as support groups and informational websites, can provide valuable insights.

Being informed enables patients to recognize symptoms early, adhere to surveillance schedules, and communicate effectively with healthcare providers. Education fosters a proactive approach to managing health, which is crucial for those with Barrett's esophagus.

Creating a Personal Action Plan for Emergencies

Developing a personal action plan for emergencies is crucial for patients with Barrett's esophagus. This plan should outline steps to take if symptoms worsen or if complications arise. Key components may include a list of emergency contacts, medications, and a description of symptoms that warrant immediate attention.

Having this plan accessible—whether saved on a phone or kept in a visible location—ensures quick access during a crisis. Sharing this plan with family members can also prepare them to assist in emergencies, making everyone more equipped to handle unexpected health challenges.

The Role of Nutrition in Recovery from Complications

Nutrition plays a vital role in recovery from complications associated with Barrett's esophagus. A balanced diet rich in fruits, vegetables, lean proteins, and whole grains can help promote healing and reduce inflammation. Avoiding trigger foods—like caffeine, alcohol, and high-fat meals—can also aid in symptom management and improve overall digestive health.

To establish a nutrition plan, consider consulting a registered dietitian who specializes in gastrointestinal health. They can provide personalized recommendations that align with your dietary preferences and medical needs, ensuring a comprehensive approach to managing Barrett's esophagus.

Support Resources for Dealing with Complications

Accessing support resources is essential for individuals managing Barrett's esophagus and its complications. Support groups, whether in-person or online, offer a platform for sharing experiences and coping strategies. These groups can help alleviate feelings of isolation and provide emotional support.

Additionally, educational resources provided by organizations specializing in gastrointestinal disorders can enhance understanding of the condition. Utilizing these resources fosters a supportive community and aids in navigating the challenges of Barrett's esophagus.

Importance of Discussing Concerns with Healthcare Providers

Open communication with healthcare providers is crucial for managing Barrett's esophagus. Patients should feel empowered to discuss any concerns or symptoms they experience. This dialogue can lead to timely interventions and adjustments in treatment plans tailored to individual needs.

Regular check-ins with your healthcare provider can also ensure that monitoring schedules and lifestyle recommendations remain aligned with your health goals. Building a strong, communicative relationship with your provider can greatly enhance your management of the condition.

Long-Term Follow-Up Care Strategies

Long-term follow-up care is essential for patients with Barrett's esophagus. Regular surveillance through endoscopy, as recommended by your healthcare provider, helps monitor any changes in the esophagus. These check-ups are crucial for early detection of complications, including dysplasia or cancer.

In addition to surveillance, lifestyle modifications—such as a healthy diet, regular exercise, and avoiding tobacco and excessive alcohol—can significantly impact long-term health outcomes. Creating a schedule for follow-ups and incorporating healthy habits into daily life will support better management of Barrett's esophagus.

Inspirational Stories of Overcoming Complications

Hearing inspirational stories from others who have successfully navigated complications related to Barrett's esophagus can be incredibly motivating. Many individuals share their journeys of overcoming health challenges through lifestyle changes, medical interventions, and support networks. These stories often highlight resilience, determination, and the importance of seeking help.

Connecting with others who have similar experiences can offer hope and practical insights into managing Barrett's esophagus. Whether through support groups or online forums, sharing stories and strategies can empower patients to take charge of their health journey.

CHAPTER 9:

Conclusion and Next Steps

Recap of Key Points Discussed in the Book

Throughout this book, we explored the essential aspects of managing Barrett's Esophagus, focusing on its causes, especially GERD, and the importance of early intervention. We emphasized dietary changes, lifestyle adjustments, and effective support strategies that can significantly improve the quality of life for those diagnosed with this condition. Understanding the role of acid reflux in the development of Barrett's Esophagus and recognizing the symptoms are crucial first steps in proactive management.

Additionally, we outlined various approaches to manage the symptoms, such as avoiding trigger foods, maintaining a healthy weight, and implementing effective stress management techniques. Engaging with healthcare providers for regular check-ups and utilizing available resources for education were highlighted as vital components in the management of Barrett's Esophagus.

Encouragement for Proactive Management of Barrett's Esophagus

Proactive management of Barrett's Esophagus involves taking control of your health through informed choices and consistent monitoring of symptoms. Implementing dietary changes, such as incorporating more fruits and vegetables while reducing processed foods, can help minimize reflux episodes. Staying educated about your condition and regularly discussing it with your healthcare provider can empower you to make necessary adjustments and seek treatments when needed.

Furthermore, establishing a routine that includes regular physical activity and stress-relief techniques, such as meditation or yoga, can significantly enhance your well-being. Recognizing the importance of prompt medical attention for any concerning symptoms will aid in preventing potential complications associated with Barrett's Esophagus.

Importance of Ongoing Education and Support

Ongoing education is crucial for anyone managing Barrett's Esophagus. Staying updated on the latest research and treatment options can lead to better outcomes. Many patients find value in joining support groups or attending workshops that focus on living with Barrett's Esophagus, where they can learn from the experiences of others and share their own journeys.

Support systems, whether they come from family, friends, or healthcare professionals, play a significant role in maintaining motivation and mental well-being. Seeking out educational materials, webinars, or local health seminars can provide continuous learning opportunities, enabling individuals to navigate their health journeys more effectively.

Overview of Resources for Continued Learning

A variety of resources are available for individuals seeking to deepen their understanding of Barrett's Esophagus. Reputable websites, such as those from the American Gastroenterological Association or the American Society for Gastrointestinal Endoscopy, offer up-to-date information and research findings. Books, online forums, and patient advocacy organizations can also be valuable sources of knowledge and support.

In addition to online resources, consider local libraries or community centers that may host informational sessions or workshops. Engaging with healthcare providers about recommended reading materials or reliable online resources can further ensure you have access to the most accurate and relevant information.

Encouragement to Engage with Healthcare Providers Regularly

Regular communication with healthcare providers is essential for managing Barrett's Esophagus effectively. Scheduling routine check-ups allows for monitoring the condition and adjusting treatment plans as needed. Be open about any symptoms or concerns, as early intervention can help prevent complications associated with Barrett's Esophagus.

Patients should feel empowered to ask questions and discuss their health actively. Building a collaborative relationship with healthcare providers fosters a supportive environment where patients can feel confident in their care decisions.

The Role of Community and Support Networks

Being part of a community or support network can significantly enhance the management of Barrett's Esophagus. These networks offer emotional support, practical advice, and a sense of belonging. Connecting with others who share similar experiences can provide insights into effective coping strategies and lifestyle changes.

Consider exploring online forums, social media groups, or local support groups dedicated to Barrett's Esophagus and related conditions. Engaging in discussions and sharing personal experiences can lead to valuable exchanges of information and encouragement.

Personalizing Health Journeys Based on Individual Needs

Every individual's health journey is unique, especially regarding Barrett's Esophagus. It's essential to personalize your approach based on specific symptoms, lifestyle, and health goals. Working closely with a healthcare provider to develop a tailored plan can ensure that dietary and lifestyle modifications align with your needs.

Listening to your body and adjusting your management strategies as necessary is key. This may involve experimenting with different diets, stress-management techniques, or medications, always under the guidance of a healthcare professional to determine what works best for you.

Importance of Maintaining a Positive Outlook

Maintaining a positive outlook can have a profound impact on managing Barrett's Esophagus. Fostering a mindset focused on resilience and adaptability can help you cope with the challenges associated with the condition. Practices such as gratitude journaling or mindfulness meditation can enhance your mental well-being and promote a healthier lifestyle.

Surrounding yourself with supportive individuals who uplift and encourage you can also contribute to a positive mindset. Celebrating small victories in your health journey, whether related to dietary changes or symptom management, helps reinforce a positive perspective.

Sharing Knowledge with Others for Mutual Benefit

Sharing knowledge about Barrett's Esophagus not only helps others but also reinforces your understanding of the condition. Engaging in discussions with peers, participating in community events, or writing articles can facilitate the exchange of information and experiences. This collaborative approach can lead to greater awareness and support for those affected by Barrett's Esophagus.

Additionally, educating family and friends can create a supportive environment that promotes healthy lifestyle choices. By sharing what you've learned, you contribute to a broader understanding of Barrett's Esophagus, ultimately benefiting the entire community.

The Evolving Understanding of Barrett's Esophagus and Research

Research into Barrett's Esophagus is continually evolving, leading to improved management strategies and potential treatment options. Keeping abreast of new studies and findings can empower patients to make informed decisions about their care. Many academic journals and healthcare organizations regularly publish updates that are accessible to patients.

Engaging with your healthcare provider about recent research and clinical trials can open up new avenues for treatment. Participating in discussions about innovative approaches or emerging therapies may enhance your management plan and ensure it aligns with the latest advancements in care.

Commitment to Health and Well-Being as a Lifelong Journey

Managing Barrett's Esophagus is a lifelong commitment that encompasses various aspects of health and wellness. Adopting a holistic approach, including balanced nutrition, regular exercise, and mental well-being, is essential. Recognizing that this is an ongoing journey encourages individuals to remain proactive in their health management.

Being committed to continuous improvement means setting realistic health goals and regularly reassessing your strategies. Establishing a routine that incorporates healthy habits can support long-term wellness and enhance the quality of life.

A Call to Action for Continued Engagement with Health and Wellness

To successfully manage Barrett's Esophagus, it's essential to engage actively with your health and wellness journey. This means being proactive in seeking out information, adjusting lifestyle choices, and connecting with healthcare professionals regularly. By taking these steps, you can stay informed and prepared to tackle any challenges that arise.

Consider setting specific goals related to diet, exercise, or support network engagement, and track your progress. This commitment to ongoing engagement can lead to better health outcomes and an improved quality of life.

Final Thoughts on Living Well with Barrett's Esophagus

Living well with Barrett's Esophagus involves a combination of informed choices, regular healthcare engagement, and support from the community. By prioritizing your health, staying educated, and fostering a positive mindset, you can effectively manage your condition and enhance your quality of life. Remember that every individual's journey is unique, and adapting strategies that resonate with your lifestyle is key to long-term success.

Common Concerns and FAQs

Common Concerns

Individuals with Barrett's Esophagus often worry about managing symptoms and the potential risks associated with their condition. Common concerns include the fear of worsening symptoms, such as increased heartburn or difficulty swallowing. It's essential to understand that proactive management can significantly alleviate these worries. This includes regular consultations with healthcare providers to adjust treatment plans and explore effective symptom relief strategies.

Patients may also be anxious about the possibility of esophageal cancer. While Barrett's Esophagus is considered a precancerous condition, many individuals live without severe complications by adhering to treatment protocols and monitoring. Staying informed and engaged in their healthcare can empower patients to navigate their concerns effectively.

What should I do if I experience severe symptoms?

If you experience severe symptoms like intense chest pain, difficulty swallowing, or significant weight loss, it's crucial to seek immediate medical attention. These symptoms may indicate complications that require urgent evaluation and intervention. In the meantime, try to keep a symptom diary to note when symptoms occur and any potential triggers, which can be valuable information for your healthcare provider.

In addition to seeking medical help, adopting lifestyle modifications can be beneficial. Elevating the head of your bed, avoiding large meals, and steering clear of known irritants, such as spicy or fatty foods, can help minimize severe symptoms. Always consult your doctor before making significant changes to your treatment plan.

How often should I have my esophagus monitored?

Monitoring frequency for Barrett's Esophagus typically depends on the severity of the condition and your individual risk factors. Most patients are advised to undergo endoscopic surveillance every 1 to 3 years, but your healthcare provider will tailor this recommendation based on your biopsy results and symptoms. It's vital to discuss your specific monitoring schedule during each appointment to ensure you receive the most appropriate care.

In preparation for these appointments, consider keeping track of any changes in your symptoms or diet that may affect your condition. This information can help your doctor make informed decisions regarding your surveillance plan and any necessary adjustments to your treatment.

Can Barrett's Esophagus lead to cancer?

Barrett's Esophagus has the potential to increase the risk of esophageal cancer, particularly if dysplasia (abnormal cell growth) is present. However, the majority of individuals with Barrett's do not develop cancer. Understanding the relationship between Barrett's and cancer is crucial for managing your health effectively. Regular monitoring and early intervention can significantly reduce this risk.

To mitigate the chances of progression to cancer, adhering to treatment plans and making lifestyle changes is essential. This includes not only medication adherence but also maintaining a healthy diet, managing GERD symptoms, and attending regular screenings as recommended by your healthcare provider.

What dietary changes are most beneficial?

A diet that minimizes acidic and spicy foods is crucial for managing Barrett's Esophagus. Focus on incorporating alkaline foods such as leafy greens, bananas, and melons, which can help neutralize stomach acid. Additionally, it's beneficial to include whole grains and lean proteins, as these are less likely to trigger reflux. Aim for smaller, more frequent meals instead of large ones to help reduce acid production.

Also, pay attention to hydration and opt for water instead of carbonated or caffeinated beverages, which can exacerbate symptoms. Keeping a food diary can assist you in identifying which foods worsen your symptoms, allowing you to tailor your diet accordingly for optimal management.

How do I cope with anxiety related to my diagnosis?

Coping with anxiety related to a Barrett's Esophagus diagnosis involves several practical strategies. First, consider seeking support from mental health professionals, such as a therapist or counselor, who can help you process your feelings and develop coping techniques. Mindfulness practices, like meditation and deep-breathing exercises, can also help reduce anxiety and improve your overall mental well-being.

Building a support network is another effective strategy. Connecting with others who have Barrett's Esophagus through support groups or online forums can provide valuable insights and emotional support. Sharing experiences and learning from others can empower you to manage your condition with greater confidence.

What is Barrett's Esophagus?

Barrett's Esophagus is a condition characterized by changes in the lining of the esophagus, often resulting from chronic acid reflux, also known as gastroesophageal reflux disease (GERD). This condition occurs when the normal squamous cells in the esophagus are replaced by columnar cells, which are more resistant to acid but can lead to complications if left untreated. Understanding this change is crucial for managing symptoms and preventing potential progression to esophageal cancer.

Awareness of Barrett's Esophagus is essential for anyone experiencing chronic heartburn or acid reflux. Early intervention can help manage symptoms effectively and monitor the condition. Regular check-ups with a healthcare provider can aid in tracking any changes and implementing necessary lifestyle adjustments to maintain esophageal health.

What are the symptoms of Barrett's Esophagus?

Common symptoms of Barrett's Esophagus include persistent heartburn, difficulty swallowing (dysphagia), chest pain, and regurgitation of food or sour liquid. Individuals may also experience a sensation of a lump in the throat, which can be uncomfortable and alarming. Recognizing these symptoms is essential for seeking timely medical evaluation and appropriate management.

If you notice these symptoms, especially if they worsen or become more frequent, consult your healthcare provider. Keeping a symptom log can help you articulate your experiences during appointments, allowing for more effective diagnosis and treatment planning tailored to your specific needs.

How is Barrett's Esophagus diagnosed?

Diagnosis of Barrett's Esophagus typically involves an endoscopy, during which a healthcare provider uses a flexible tube with a camera to visualize the esophagus. If abnormal cells are suspected, a biopsy will be performed to assess the cellular changes more closely. This process is critical for confirming Barrett's and determining the appropriate management plan.

To prepare for an endoscopy, your doctor may advise fasting for several hours beforehand. It's also helpful to discuss any medications you're taking, as some may need to be paused prior to the procedure. Understanding this diagnostic process can alleviate some anxiety and help you feel more prepared for your appointment.

What dietary changes should I make?

To manage Barrett's Esophagus effectively, focus on dietary changes that minimize acid reflux. Prioritize a diet rich in whole foods, including plenty of fruits, vegetables, and whole grains, while limiting processed foods high in fat and sugar. Avoid trigger foods such as citrus fruits, tomatoes, chocolate, and spicy dishes, which can exacerbate symptoms.

Incorporate smaller, balanced meals throughout the day rather than a few large meals. This approach can help prevent excessive acid production. Keeping a food diary can assist you in identifying and eliminating foods that worsen your symptoms, allowing for a more tailored and effective dietary plan.

Can Barrett's Esophagus be reversed?

While Barrett's Esophagus damage may not be completely reversible, early intervention can effectively manage symptoms and reduce associated risks. Regular monitoring and appropriate lifestyle changes, such as medication adherence and dietary adjustments, can stabilize the condition and improve quality of life. Engaging actively in your healthcare plan is vital to achieving the best outcomes.

Staying informed about your condition and making proactive health choices can empower you to manage Barrett's Esophagus effectively. Consult your healthcare provider about available treatment options and lifestyle strategies that can help mitigate symptoms and prevent progression.